CHILDREN'S AILMENTS

CHILDREN'S AILMENTS

Dr D G Delvin

MB BS LRCP MRCS DOBST
RCOG DCH FPA CERT
MRCGP DIP VEN

The ROYAL
SOCIETY of
MEDICINE

SUNBURST BOOKS

Editorial Advisor

DR KATHARINE A ORTON
MB BS MRCGP
DCH DRCOG

This edition first published in 1995 by
Sunburst Books, Deacon House,
65 Old Church Street, London SW3 5BS.

ISBN 1 85778 162 7

Printed and bound in China

INTRODUCTION

I hope you find our quick reference guide to childhood ailments a help to you in bringing up your youngsters and maintaining their health.

All children become ill sometimes, and this little book will help you to understand the common problems which may happen to your boy or girl.

Dr David Delvin

WARNING

No book can ever replace the advice and care of a physician.
So, please: if you are in any doubt about whether your child's symptoms are dangerous or not, ***always contact your own family doctor*** (or other suitably qualified health professional).

Children can become extremely ill with alarming speed. Therefore, please do remember that a quick telephone call for medical advice may save a boy or girl's life.

ABDOMINAL PAIN *(see **Tummy Ache**)*

ABRASIONS *(see **Grazes**)*

ABSCESS

Abscesses are collections of pus. In childhood a common site is on the gums. These dental abscesses are caused when an infection gets into the gums through decayed teeth.

The classic symptom of a dental abscess is a painful swelling which develops quite suddenly on the gum. The only remedy is to take the child to a dentist as soon as possible. The dentist will drain the abscess and may also remove the tooth that intially caused the problem.

ADENOIDS

All children have adenoids. The only trouble is that in some youngsters the adenoids grow too big and may cause problems with breathing, which in turn may cause snoring.

The adenoids are small pads of gland tissue which are found at the back of the cavity of your child's nose, just above her palate. They are usually quite large in young children, so they may obstruct the passage of air through the cavity at the back of the nose. If they get very big, then the child will tend to snore a lot and to speak with a 'blocked up' sort of voice.

A lot of youngsters grow out of this phase without any treatment. However, others have to have their adenoids removed. This is an operation that is usually performed at the same time the tonsils are taken out.

ALLERGIES

Many children are allergic to such things as pollen, animal hairs, tiny mites in house dust, feathers, drugs or food colourings.

Symptoms which allergies produce are variable, but common manifestations include asthma, hay fever, some types of eczema and dermatitis, and urticaria (nettle rash). Very occasionally allergies may even cause the child to collapse and even become unconscious.

What happens in an allergic reaction? The child's body is exposed to an agent called an antigen. Although this antigen does not produce any obvious ill effects on the first occasion, the child's tissues produce substances called antibodies in response. On the next occasion that his body is exposed to the same antigen (whether it's grass or tree pollen, animal hair or skin scales or some type of food), the union of antigen and antibody is liable to produce dramatic effects, such as a severe skin rash, an asthma attack or a bout similar to those of hay fever symptoms.

In many families there is a marked inherited tendency to allergic conditions – particularly eczema, hay fever, dust-mite allergy and asthma. Happily, new methods of treatment are making things easier for the allergic child. These include newer antihistamine drugs (which do not cause sedation, like the old antihistamines), and other methods to protect the child's body tissues against allergies.

ALOPECIA

Alopecia just means baldness. Unfortunately, a few children (for reasons which are not understood) develop unusual forms of childhood baldness. One form is called alopecia areata, and the other is called alopecia totalis.

Alopecia areata is much more common. In this condition there are only small localised patches of hair loss. Fortunately, in many children the hair regrows after a few months. It's important to distinguish this condition from ringworm, which quite often gives a similar appearance.

Alopecia totalis is fortunately rare. It results in loss of all the hair on the head, often including the eyebrows. A typical case was that of the famous swimmer Duncan Goodhew.

Unfortunately, the cause of the condition is not known, and the outlook for regrowth of hair is not all that good.

ANAEMIA (ANEMIA)

Anaemia means weakness of the blood. This is usually due to lack of iron, but can have other causes. Lack of iron can be caused by:

* Inadequate intake of iron in food

* Loss of iron because of bleeding

Anaemia is not very common in children, but iron-deficiency anaemia does occur in some babies and toddlers, as both breast milk and cow's milk are lacking in iron. A healthy full-term baby has acquired from its mother enough iron stores to last him for the first six months of life. However, if his mother was anaemic during pregnancy, he may not have obtained enough iron from her.

The same thing may happen with premature babies, and with twins, who have to share their mother's iron between them. In children, iron deficiency may be caused by a diet lacking in iron, so there is every reason to encourage youngsters to eat meat and fish, which are rich in this mineral. Contrary to common belief, spinach is not a particularly good source of iron.

The symptoms of anaemia are paleness, fatigue and, sometimes, breathlessness. Some children have an odd tendency to eat strange 'foods' such as ice cubes. The treatment of iron-deficiency anaemia is to replace the iron with iron-containing medicines. The results of this treatment are very good indeed.

For other occasional causes of anaemia see **Sickle Cell Disease** and **Leukaemia**.

APPENDICITIS

Appendicitis means inflammation of the appendix – a small organ located in the lower right-hand corner of the stomach. The cause is unknown.

There's about a one in ten chance that your child will have his appendix removed one day. So this operation, which is called 'appendicectomy' (or 'appendectomy' if you are American), is one of the most common of all surgical procedures. Appendix removal is a very safe operation, though all 'ops' do of course carry a slight risk. If your child gets appendicitis one day, there is no need for you to worry, since he's almost certain to have a good recovery.

The classic symptoms are as follows:

* Tummy pain increasing over several hours

* Loss of interest in food

* Vomiting – but very rarely more than once

* A very off-colour feeling

* A moderately raised temperature

If your child has a tummy-ache which has gone on for several hours, always ring your doctor for advice.

If your GP thinks that the child might have acute appendicitis, she'll get him into hospital. Once there, he'll be examined again.

In fact, by the time a child is settled down into a hospital bed, the pain which was thought to have been caused by appendicitis will very often have disappeared so there is no need to operate.

If your child really has got acute appendicitis, he'll be taken to the operating theatre, gently eased off to sleep by the anaesthetist, and then operated on. The surgeon makes a tiny incision, removes the appendix, and then stitches up the incision. In most cases, the child should be out of hospital within a few days.

ASPIRIN
Do **not** give aspirin to your child unless your family doctor says that there are strong reasons for doing so. For the reasons why, refer to **Reye's syndrome.**

ASTHMA
This is a common chest disorder in childhood, and it's becoming commoner, perhaps because of air pollution. It is characterised by intermittent bouts of wheezing, coughing and breathlessness,

which are caused by the temporary narrowing of air passages leading to the lungs, and also to partial blockage of these passages by mucus or inflammatory swelling.

What causes asthma? There are three principal factors: an allergy, infection and stress, of which the first is by far the most important. Infection plays a modest part, and fortunately stress is a very minor one.

Allergy is an irrational defence reaction by the body to some outside stimulus: a protective response gone wrong, in fact. The child comes in contact with something tow which he is allergic and his air passages start closing down almost as if making a desperate attempt to keep out the foreign material.

If your child has asthma, you can begin by trying to identify the allergen. You may not succeed, but it's worth a try. Pollen, house dust, the dander (shed skin cells) from animals and moulds are all possible causes. And these are causes which you can do something about by keeping the child away from them. In very severe cases where there is no other solution, it may even be necessary to move to a house with less dust.

In the last few years, it's become apparent that certain foods can sometimes provoke allergy and hence asthma attacks. These include milk, eggs, cheese, coffee and food additives such as the yellow dye called tartrazine. Your family doctor or a specialist can advise you about what items of food to exclude from your child's diet to try to find out what's provoking the attacks.

Unfortunately, identifying the allergen is largely a question of trial and error. Skin tests for allergy can be arranged at special centres but they aren't all that reliable. Home trial and error is often just as good. For instance, if a girl is always sneezy when she wakes up in her bedroom but fine when she's out in the open air, it's likely that she's allergic to house dust.

Drug therapy Modern therapy is very effective, but must be closely supervised by a doctor. She will wish to adjust the treatment regularly, taking into account how severe the child's symptoms are. Another important guideline is provided by the youngster's 'Peak Flow Rate' or 'PFR', which is measured regularly, using a simple device which she blows into.

The drugs which are available include:

  * Bronchodilators. These widen the child's airways making it easier for her breath to move in and out

  * Preventers. These are drugs which reduce the swelling and mucus in the child's airways,

  * Protectors. These are longer-acting medicines, which must be taken regularly in order to keep the air passages open.

Please note that neither the preventers nor the protectors can be used to treat a sudden attack.

Attacks must be treated very promptly by bronchodilators or by steroids given orally.

  * Steroids. These are very powerful anti-inflammatory agents which can 'damp down' the wild allergic reaction of asthma. In a crisis they are often life-saving.

However, they can have potentially serious side-effects (including stunting the child's growth), so most children aren't given them long-term but only when they are really necessary.

ATHLETE'S FOOT

This is a fungus infection of the skin, which is very common among older children, especially boys. It spreads rapidly among youngsters who go barefoot on moist floors. It is often picked up in showers, changing rooms, bathrooms, school dormitories, and so on.

The fungus almost invariably attacks the gap between the fourth and the fifth toe, although it may spread to other areas.

There is really not a lot of point in taking your child to the doctor if he gets athlete's foot, since your chemist can sell you perfectly satisfactory anti-fungus creams. If these are used regularly and as directed they will control the infection.

AUTISM

Autism is an uncommon but extremely distressing disorder, in which a child seems to live in a world of his own.

The cause, unfortunately, is unknown. Parents tend to blame themselves when they have an autistic child, but this isn't justifiable. No one has the faintest idea what causes this sad condition.

The characteristic thing about the autistic child is his aloofness from other people; he really wants nothing whatever to do with them. He usualy shows no love for his parents nor for anyone else, and takes no pleasure in other people's company. This isn't his fault in any way. There is no medicine which will cure autism. The main hope is to educate the child to achieve a more normal method of behaviour. To do this, you will need the help of a child development unit with staff who are experienced in dealing with autism. Therapists usually attempt to find some way of establishing contact with the autistic child, which will be very difficult. Speech therapy is also a very important part of treatment.

The strain on the parents of an autistic child is invariably enormous. So it is very important that the family should be offered the help of a trained and sympathetic counsellor.

BED-WETTING

Bed-wetting (or nocturnal enuresis) causes both children and parents a great deal of grief.

This is a pity, because this tension and trauma is usually quite unnecessary; very often dads and mums expect far too much of their children in the matter of dryness at night.

If your child is dry at night at the age of two, then you're very lucky – and he's very unusual. But even at the age of four, half of all youngsters will still sometimes wet during the night. And a very large proportion of five-year-olds are still wet: this is natural for them.

Only after the age of five is there any point in seeking medical treatment for bed-wetting. Yet large numbers of parents of two- or-three-year-old children take them to the doctor and demand powerful (and dangerous) medicines in an effort to make their children dry.

But what about children of five-and-a-half, six or seven who keep wetting? Clearly, you have to take some action about this.

First, don't assume, as so many people do, that drugs are the answer. The drugs which are used in an effort to combat bed-wetting are not very effective – and they are actually the powerful mind-affecting agents which many adults take for depression.

The most worrying thing about these drugs is that they're supplied as pleasant-tasting fruit-flavoured syrups. So it is not surprising that a child sometimes gets at them and has an extra swig. Yet such drugs can kill.

A 'star chart' is a form of encouragement trick which has become popular in recent years. Every time he's dry the child can stick a gold star on a large calendar in his room.

If you do use the star chart, make sure that you don't make the child feel a failure every time he's wet. Also, you must take care that his friends don't see your child's chart and so realise the he has this problem. Children can really be very cruel about this sort of thing.

The best way of treating bed-wetting it to use an alarm, an entirely safe device that works by means of a special electrical pad under your child's sheet. If he passes just the tiniest drop of urine during the night, that drop will complete an electrical circuit which runs through the pad. It's a bit like the pad of a burglar alarm, in fact. The battery-powered circuit is connected to a buzzer which is placed by his bed, and the completion of the circuit sets off the buzzer – and it's so loud that it will wake any child. Naturally, you will have told the youngster that he's to get up and go to the toilet as soon as he hears the buzzer.

In a majority of cases this treatment will cure the child of bed-wetting within a few months. It can't cure all cases, but it is often successful where drugs and star charts have failed. And there are no side-effects.

Remember that a number of children who wet the bed do so because of some emotional problem. They may be worried about a bully at school, or about rows at home; but, without meaning to, they respond to whatever psychological stress is affecting them by wetting themselves at night.

If your child has been dry for a year or two but then inexplicably becomes wet again, it is likely that this is due to some form of psychological stress. Obviously, you owe it to him to try to find out what it is.

Finally, an appreciable proportion of children who are very late bed-wetters do turn out to have some internal structural abnormality of their urinary system, and sometimes have a urinary infection (see **Urinary Infections**).

BEE STINGS (see *Stings*)

BIRTHMARKS

Nearly all children have some sort of mark on the skin at birth. Fortunately, well over 90 per cent of these marks are so small or are so unnoticeable that they do not cause any distress. Many of the rest are only a centimetre or two across, and are on parts of the body where they do not matter very much.

However, about 5 children in 100 do have bigger

marks (or marks on the face) which cause both them and their parents a lot of distress. Happily, some types of birthmarks do shrink in the first few years of life; your GP or child health clinic doctor may be able to reassure you that your child has this type of shrinking mark. If this is the case, no further treatment will be needed.

If not do your level best not to 'go on' about the mark within earshot of the child. Also, reassure her that, although it is noticeable, it doesn't make her different from anyone else, or inferior in any way – and that you love her just the same.

Many marks can be dealt with by laser treatment, or by surgery, or by camouflage with make-up. However, you may well find that your doctor is not keen to rush into surgery or laser therapy, for several reasons.

First, as the birthmark might shrink right down, treatment may not be needed at all. Second, a small child is usually difficult to operate on from a technical point of view. The bigger she gets, the easier it is to refashion the blemished area of her skin. So again, the surgeon may prefer to delay as long as possible. Third, doctors do realise that there is a small risk from any form of treatment.

If surgical or laser treatment isn't practical for your child at the moment, then it is well worth using one of the special 'camouflage' make-ups which are specifically designed to disguise birth-marks. They come in a variety of skin tints, so you should be able to match the skin colour.

BLEEDING
In cases of heavy bleeding, the one really vital thing is immediately to press something (a clean

cloth is preferable) really firmly on to the child's bleeding point. Keep pressing – and do not let up untill expert help arrives.

Never apply a tourniquets, as this is liable to cause gangrene, which could result in the child losing a limb.

BOILS

A boil occurs when a germ, the scientific name of which is *Staphylococcus aureus,* gets into a little follicle (pit) in the skin, and produces pus.

Treatment of boils is a bit unsatisfactory. Some doctors prescribe antibiotics, but it's doubtful whether the antibiotic can really penetrate the 'wall' around the boil and do any good.

The traditional treatment of trying to 'draw' the boil with magnesium sulphate paste is probably as good as anything, and will do no harm.

A boil which has actually developed a head on it can often be lanced by your doctor. What you should *not* do is to squeeze the boil yourself – this is likely to spread germs to other parts of his skin (and possibly to you as well).

Many children get recurrent boils, especially if they're run down. If your youngster frequently gets boils, then you should take her to the doctor. Take along a specimen of urine, so that the doctor can check it for sugar. This is because recurrent boils may indicate diabetes.

BOWEL PROBLEMS

There are two types of bowel problems which are common in childhood and which may cause parents some degree of concern: these two are diarrhoea and constipation .

Constipation This means an inability to pass bowel motions as often as desired. Unfortunately, that's a very relative expression. In other words, if you think your child should have his bowels open every day, then you're going to regard a child who has a three-times-a-week bowel action as having constipation.

If you couldn't care less how often your youngster has his bowels open, then you won't regard three times a week (or even once a week) as being constipation. If you take the view that it doesn't matter to his health, you'd be right.

If you find it hard to accept that children should be allowed to pass a motion as and when they want to – not on a rigidly laid-down schedule – then instead of laxatives, just give your family lots of fruit and vegetables.

Fruit and veg are full of fibre, which stimulates the bowel to work naturally. So too is bran, but don't get carried away with the current fashion: if you give really massive doses of fibre in the form of bran you can actually produce a blockage of the bowels.

Finally, ignore the persistent urgings of others who say: 'But it's not right, dear: he hasn't been today.' He'll survive.

Diarrhoea Unfortunately every parent is all too familiar with the fact that children do tend to have diarrhoea at times – and often in the most wildly inconvenient and embarrassing places (such as aeroplanes, or on the motorway). Let's look at the possible causes.

Diarrhoea in young babies is a very common symptom, and often one of little significance, but if it persists it is best dealt with by the family doctor. In some babies, diarrhoea is simply a reaction to too much sugar in a bottlefeed. In a very small proportion of children, it may indicate some important underlying disorder, for example coeliac disease *(see **Coeliac Disease**).*

Diarrhoea in older babies, toddlers or children can occasionally be casued by cystic fibrosis *(see **Cystic Fibrosis**)* or other serious conditions, but it is much more likely to be part of infectious diarrhoea and vomiting (D&V), which will affect nearly all families at some time or another.

Very often, several members of the family get it at once, or one after the other. And often it's the young children who suffer most. This is because the fluid loss caused by an attack of D&V can be very much more serious for a tiny child, whose fluid reserves are much smaller than those of a grown-up. An attack in a young baby can have devastating consequences, as severe dehydration (that is, a lack of fluid) can result in death with alarming speed. Admittedly, most bouts of D&V are not serious – but never regard diarrhoea or vomiting in a baby as something trivial. If you are in any real doubt, ask your doctor for advice.

Most cases of D&V are caused by infection, with small germs which are all too readily spread from one human being to another. That is why D&V so often spreads through a family.

D&V starts with someone who may or may not feel ill but is excreting the germs in his or her bowel motions. If a germ from this person's bowel motions gets into someone else's food or drink, then down they go with the 'bug'.

Here are a few basic rules for prevention of D&V in the home. It is impossible to rule out all attacks, but you can cut the chances of D&V occurring to a minimum by following these health principles:

* Make sure that all members of your family wash their hands after passing a bowel motion

* Try to get your family to wash their hands before meals – a quick rinse is sufficient

* Ensure that anyone who is preparing food or babies' bottles washes their hands first

* Make sure that all frozen food, particularly **poultry**, is thoroughly defrosted

* Don't let anyone who has boils on their hands, or a septic finger, prepare food or babies' bottles

* Breast-feed your baby if possible. It's so very easy for bottles and teats to be contaminated by germs

As mentioned earlier, babies can get seriously dehydrated by diarrhoea or vomiting. So, in the case of a young baby, don't hesitate to seek medical advice.

Your GP will probably prescribe a powder rich in minerals, to which you add boiled water.

Antibiotics such as penicillin will *not* help. Most D&V infections are caused by viruses – and viruses are the type of germs which are not affected by antibiotics. Indeed, some cases of diarrhoea can actually be made worse by antibiotics.

While the child is on the boiled water mixture, don't succumb to the temptationion to give solids, or even milk. This is probably one of the commonest causes of a relapse of symptoms.

In really desperate cases of D&V, your GP will arrange admission to hospital. But in the average case, your child's own defences against infection will enable him to defeat the infection after a couple of days provided that he gets enough fluid (i.e. the boiled water mixture).

BREATH-HOLDING ATTACKS

Some small children respond to emotional stress by simply gritting their teeth and refusing to breathe. After a minute or so they become blue in the face and may even lose consciousness. Should this happen, don't panic; as soon as the child is unconsious he'll breathe normally again.

This symptom is very alarming for the parents. Difficult though it may be to manage, an attitude of calmness and sympathy will give the best results. All children who suffer from breath-holding attacks grow out of them with time.

BRONCHITIS

Children **do** get bronchitis, but this is a different condition from the chronic (long-term) disease of adults. In children, bronchitis is an acute (short-term) condition caused by a virus.

Bronchitis actually means inflammation of the tubes leading to the lungs. In children, it may occur as a complication of colds, 'flu and other virus infections. The child gets tightness of the chest associated with a dry, painful cough. Later, a good deal of yellow sputum may be produced. If you suspect bronchitis, call your GP, who may or may not prescribe antibiotics. In most cases, the child will make a full recovery.

BRONCHIOLITIS

A virus infection common in very young children in winter. Usually a cold progresses to wheezing and/or difficulty in breathing. If this happens ***ring your GP at once***. Some children need to be taken to hospital for oxygen treatment.

BRUISES

Most bruises are best left untreated. However, applying ice wrapped in a towel can help, and a cold compress will help in relieving pain. Painful or extensive bruising should seen by your GP, who make sure there are no other injuries.

BURNS AND SCALDS

The moment you realise a child has been burned (or scalded), drench the affected part in cold water immediately. If there are smouldering clothes on the skin, cut them off before they do more damage.

Remove any bangles or rings, as the skin beneath and around them may start to swell up.

In the case of a large burn, don't apply anything: cover the affected area with a very clean cloth, and get the child to medical help.

In the case of a very small burn, you can safely apply any of the standard antiseptic creams.

C.F. *(see **Cystic Fibrosis**)*

CANCER

Fortunately, cancer is quite rare in childhood, so it is unlikely that you will have to face the appalling ordeal of having to look after a much loved child with this condition.

The only relatively common cancers in children are leukaemia, Hodgkin's disease, lymphoma, Wilm's tumour and neuroblastoma.

Leukaemia is a cancer of the blood, and of the cells which manufacture the blood *(see **Leukaemia**)*.

Hodgkin's disease is a much milder cancer (in that the outlook is generally fairly good these days), which affects the child's lymph glands and makes them swell up painlessly.

Treatment with anti-cancer drugs gives very good results. Lymphoma is a very similar condition.

Wilm's tumour (nephroblastoma) is a form of cancer that affects the child's kidney. The main symptom which it produces is that of a rapidly-growing abdominal swelling; as soon as the doctor has made the diagnosis, the tumour must be removed surgically. This is the only way to save the child's life.

Neuroblastoma is a cancer of the child's adrenal gland, which is located just above the kidney.

Again, the main symptom is a rapidly growing abdominal swelling. Surgical removal, which is often combined with radiotherapy, is the best hope of cure for this type of cancer.

The outlook in most types of childhood cancer has improved a good deal in recent years.

CAR SICKNESS

Car sickness is very common, very trying, and can be very messy. Good preventive measures are as follows:

1 Don't suggest to the child that he will probably be ill

2 Give him lots of mental games to play so that you occupy his attention

3 On long journeys, consider giving a sickness-prone child an anti-sickness pill; administer the pill at least an hour before you leave

4 Make sure you have several strong plastic bags, plus baby wipes or some similar preparations for cleaning up

CARBON MONOXIDE POISONING (see **Gas Poisoning**)

CATARRH

This means the accumulation of mucus in the air spaces behind your child's nose, so that it blocks up the air passages, so it is difficult to breathe.

Unfortunately, it may get into the tubes which lead from his throat to his ears – making him (at least temporarily) deaf. It increases the chance of ear aches (see **Ear Ache**). And it may well drip down into his throat and from there to the tubes leading into his lungs, causing coughing.

The sort of things that provoke catarrh are air pollutants (especially cigarette smoke), dust, pollen and germs. When children are very young, they are exposed to a barrage of such attacks –

and their mucous membranes almost invariably respond by producing catarrh. As they get older, children become relatively more resistant to these attacks, but children with allergies may continue to have problems with catarrh. There is, unfortunately, no medicine which makes catarrh instantly go away. All your doctor can do is to give you something to help the symptoms; he can't produce an instant cure. Among the things he's likely to prescribe are:

* Nose drops, which are helpful if used for a few days – especially if given to a baby half an hour before feeds so that he isn't all snuffly when he's trying to swallow. *Note:* prolonged use of these drops can damage the nose, so your doctor will usually advise giving them for four or five days only

* Inhalants, which are often soothing and comforting to a child. Old-fashioned inhalants can be bought reasonably cheaply over the counter from a chemist and are quite effective for temporary relief of symptoms

* Antihistamines, which are anti-allergy drugs. These are of some value where there seems to be a definite element of allergy involved in the child's catarrh

There are also other measures you can take to help a child with bad catarrh. First, try cutting down on the irritants to which her nose is exposed, in particular, any dust in her bedroom. Second, avoid smoking in the house. Third, try taking her outside into the open air as much as possible, preferably into the countryside. Country air is fairly free of pollutants (even today) and just a few hours spent in the country will give a child's respiratory passages a rest from contaminants which provoke bouts of catarrh.

CEREBRAL PALSY (CP)

'Palsy' means 'paralysis', and 'cerebral' means 'to do with the brain'. So 'CP' means paralysis caused by brain injury. It usually occurs in the mother's womb or at childbirth.

The symptoms depend on which part of the child's brain has been affected. But in all cases, movement of the child's limbs and/or face is affected in some way.

There may also be involuntary movements or co-ordination problems, particularly with speech. In some cerebral palsy children, there may also be difficulties with epilepsy *(see **Epilepsy**),* blindness or deafness. Also, some children are mentally handicapped.

However it is vital to understand that many of the children with cerebral palsy do have perfectly normal intelligence.

Drugs cannot cure cerebral palsy, and they play little or no part in treatment. What is needed is very intensive education of the child's brain to help her cope with the skills of life, particularly with communicating with other people.

Physiotherapy, occupational and speech therapy and other specialised teaching all play a part. But most of the burden still falls on the parents. Their efforts in helping the child 'stretch' herself and in providing as happy and stable a home life as possible are of enormous importance to her future development.

CHICKENPOX

This is a common and usually harmless infection.
At present there is no vaccine against it.
The virus which causes chickenpox circulates in
the community, flaring up and causing outbreaks
every now and again.

Children are infectious for a day or two before the
rash appears and a week or so afterwards.
Chickenpox takes about 16 days to develop,
although a child may take between 12 and 21
days to come out in spots after exposure.

Spots develop on the trunk and on the face; they
appear as little reddish lumps, many of which
have blisters of fluid in the centre. The blisters
turn into crusts and come off after a few days.
Chickenpox spots itch like madand it's difficult
for a child to learn not to scratch.

If she's small you may find it helpful to put her in
light mittens. Keep her nails short and well-
trimmed, and make sure that they are clean to
reduce the chance of introducing germs into the
blisters. Calamine lotion, dabbed on with cotton
wool, helps relieve itching. If that doesn't work try
sitting her in a moderately warm bath into which
you have put two cupfuls of bicarbonate of soda.
Don't give aspirin.

The patient should stay in bed for a couple of
days, but after that she can run about the house
or go into the garden. There is usually no need to
call the doctor unless you are in doubt about the
diagnosis. Don't take your child to your GP's
surgery – it just leads to chickenpox being
passed to other people.

Your child shouldn't go to playgroup or school
until about 10 days after the spots appear. If

there are still scabs present give your doctor a ring to check that it is all right to send her back.

Should your child get confused or inexplicably drowsy or have fits while she has chickenpox, contact your GP right away, as these symptoms indicate that the virus is has begun to affec the nervous system. This is a rare complication which needs urgent hospital treatment. *(See **Reye's syndrome**)*.

CIRCUMCISION
Operation of removal of the foreskin, now only carried out on a small minority of boys in most Western countries (but performed routinely in Moslem and Jewish cultures).

The reason for the decline of circumcision in the West in recent years is the realisation by doctors that the operation carries appreciable risks, and no clear benefits - except in rare cases of urinary obstruction by a tight foreskin.

Circumcision is also applied to a procedure which is sometimes caried out on young girls in Africa and elsewhere. It varies in nature, but often involves removal of the clitoris and the labia (vaginal lips). This operation is of doubtful legality in western countires; for instance, a doctor who carried it out in Britain would be in difficulties with the General Medical Council.

CLEFT PALATE AND HARE LIP
To discover that your child has a cleft palate or a hare lip is a terrible shock. But both conditions can be very successfully treated these days. In fact, they are closely linked. To understand what cleft palate and hare lip are, let's look at the way

in which the baby develops while it is inside the mother's womb.

The nose, upper lip and palate are formed by three processes which grow downward from the area where the eyes are forming. When these three downward projections reach the zone where the mouth will be, they fuse together. The two lines of fusion are roughly in alignment with where the nostrils will form.

Sadly, it often happens that something goes wrong with this delicate fusion. If the projections don't join at the front, then the result will be a hare lip. If they don't join at the back, the baby will have a cleft palate.

Now you can probably see from this why a hare lip doesn't occur exactly in the middle of the upper lip, like the lip of a hare or cat. In fact, it occurs slightly to one side, just under the nostril.

And if the baby is unlucky, he may have a hare lip on both sides, with just a projection of tissue about a centimetre or so wide under the nose, between the two gaps.

Why do these problems occur? We don't know. But the important thing to appreciate is that these days it's fairly easy for a skilled paediatric surgeon to operate on a child with a hare lip or cleft palate, and to close the gap perfectly.

COELIAC DISEASE
Pronounced SEAL-ee-ack disease, this is a fairly common childhood disorder in which an abnormal sensitivity to a protein called gluten which is present in some foods prevents the child from absorbing nutrition properly from her intestine. The

result may be recurrent illness and failure to gain weight. Characteristically, the child passes large, pale bowel motions.

The condition is usually diagnosed by examining a tiny sample of the intestine under a microscope.

Once the diagnosis has been made, the child will have to go on a permanent gluten-free diet, which means excluding any products made from wheat, rye, barley and, perhaps, oats. In many countries packets containing foods suitable for coeliac patients are marked with a special symbol.

COLDS
Colds are caused by viruses, which are spread from person to person through tiny droplets breathed out from the nose and mouth. The virus can also be passed on by hand contact with another human.

Most children will get about two colds per year. If your child seems to have a lot more than that, check with your doctor.

Colds cannot be treated with penicillin or other antibiotics. So all you can do is try to ease your child's symptoms by giving her paracetamol (**DO NOT** give **aspirin**) and plenty of nice, soothing drinks. Keep her away from school or nursery until she has stopped snuffling and sneezing so the risk of infecting others is minimised.

COLIC
This is a mysterious but common condition which makes young babies scream and draw up their legs as though they are suffering from severe abdominal pain.

Rather surprisingly, doctors still don't know what causes it. Many parents continue to think that colic is caused by 'wind', but there has never been any proof of this.

If your baby gets what appears to be colic, your doctor will first want to make sure that there is nothing else wrong. Your health visitor may be able to help by suggesting adjustments to the baby's feeds and feeding routine.

But, to be honest, it is possible that nothing can be done, and that you will just have to wait till the attacks of colic stop, which they almost invariably do after about three months.

CONGENITAL DISLOCATION OF THE HIP

Congenital dislocation of the hip (CDH) is quite common. At one time it crippled many children. Today, provided that the disorder is detected early enough and treated, this should not happen.

When a newborn baby leaves hospital, one of the doctors should carry out a routine check of the baby's hips. If CDH isn't noticed before the baby leaves the hospital, there's a good chance that the problem will be picked up at your local health clinic. Once the disorder has been diagnosed, then it can be cured.

This is achieved by putting the child's legs in a special 'splint', which holds the legs apart for several months.

CONJUNCTIVITIS

This is inflammation of the 'white' of the child's eye, caused by infection or (occasionally) by a blow. The chief symptom is yellow matter coming from the eyes, especially in the morning.

An antibiotic eye ointment or drops should quickly cure the problem.

CONSTIPATION (see **Bowel Problems**)

CONVULSIONS (see **Epilepsy** and also **Feverish Convulsions**)

COUGH
All youngsters get a cough from time to time. Here are the common causes:

* Chest infections

* Catarrh

* Asthma

* Colds in which there is a lot of material dripping down the back of the throat

* Tonsillitis

Rarer and more serious causes include whooping cough, inhaled foreign bodies, and TB.

Contact a health professional for advice if a cough is causing distress, or if it goes on for more than three days.

CROUP
This word means harsh, noisy breathing, as a result of some obstruction of the child's voice-box

(larynx) and is commonly caused by infection. If it occurs, always seek medical advice - fast.

CUTS

If your child cuts herself, the first thing to do is reassure her. The next step is to control any bleeding (see **Bleeding**). Then wash the injury with soap and warm water. Dry, and apply a plaster. If a cut is deep or dirty, seek medical advice.

CYSTIC FIBROSIS

Cystic fibrosis (or fibrocystic disease) is an inherited condition which occurs about once in every 2000 births. One out of every twenty adults is a hidden carrier of the gene.

Also known as CF or mucoviscidosis, this is a disease in which the mucus produced by certain organs of the body is far thicker and more viscid than normal. The affected organs may include the lungs and pancreas.

Because CF is caused by an inherited faulty gene, there is sometimes a history of another affected child in the family. This may help to give a clue to the diagnosis.

CF tends to show itself in one of three ways:

* Recurrent chest infections. The production of thick mucus in the lungs may give the baby or toddler recurring and severe bouts of coughing and wheezing

* Blockage of the intestines in the new born. This occurs because the disease has hit the pancreas, which cannot therefore produce the juices which digest food

* Frequent passing of large, pale bowel
  motions – also caused by a lack of the
  essential digestive juices

This is a very serious disease. But the outlook
has improved quite a bit in recent years,
especially since the CF gene was discovered in
1989, opening up the prospect of widespread
screening and gene therapy.

Treatment may include antibiotics to control lung
infections, aerosol inhalations, drugs to 'thin out'
thick mucus, drugs to open up the air passages,
administration of oxygen, physiotherapy, vitamin
supplements, and enzyme preparations which
help replace the missing pancreatic juices.

Unfortunately, the enzymes may have side-effects
when administered in high dosage, so get your
GP's up-to-date advice about them.

A system of breathing called FET (Forced
Expiration Technique) is taught by physiothera-
pists and is of great help to children who are old
enough to learn it.

DEAFNESS

If you suspect your child may be even slightly
deaf, you should have her hearing checked
urgently.

If deafness is not diagnosed promptly (and if
appropriate action is not taken), it is almost
certain that an enormous amount of harm will be
done to the affected child's educational, social
and emotional development.

Unfortunately, it still quite often happens that a
baby is *not* diagnosed as being wholly or partly

deaf. By the time anybody finds out, she may have dropped far behind other children in her age group in acquiring linguistic and other skills. You can imagine the damage that this may cause.

In fact, deafness ought to be picked up at the routine hearing checks given in infancy – and in many cases, it is. Treatment and/or special help with speech can then be started.

There are many possible causes of childhood deafness, including German measles contracted during pregnancy; meningitis and recurrent ear infections. Temporary deafness may accompany ear ache *(see **Ear Ache**)*. Sadly, in many cases we don't know why a child is born deaf.

DIABETES

Diabetes in childhood is common. It used to be a death sentence, until the day in the 1920s when two young Canadian researchers managed to save a diabetic boy's life with the revolutionary new treatment of insulin – a hormone which in those early days had to be extracted from the pancreas of animals. From that time onwards it has been possible for all children who suffer from diabetes to survive and to live normal and healthy lives.

To understand diabetes, you have to appreciate that the human body runs on fuel - and its fuel is glucose. Glucose is like the petrol that runs most motor vehicles. A great deal of the food which you eat is broken down into glucose by your digestive system, so that it can be used by your body as fuel.

In the same way as cars won't work unless there is a spark of electricity to help burn the petrol, the body's glucose can't be burned unless there is something to help it burn – and that something else is called insulin.

You have plenty of insulin in your body. It is a chemical produced by your pancreas, a gland located near your stomach.

In children the pancreas does not function properly. We still don't really understand why, but the result is that not enough insulin is produced to burn up the body's glucose. If the body fails to produce sufficient insulin for its needs then the level of glucose in the body starts to rise.

Soon there is so much glucose in the body that the only way to get rid of it is by passing it out in the urine. That is why one of the most important warning signs of this disease is a tendency to pass large quantities of urine. Other prominent symptoms are extreme thirst and marked weight loss. Some children also get a lot of boils.

So any child who has any of the above symptoms should certainly be taken to his GP, who will test the urine for glucose.

If the test is positive, this is an indication of diabetes – although further investigations will probably be necessary to confirm the diagnosis.

If your child has got diabetes, it is bound to come as a shock. You may not even be able to take all of it in to begin with.

But take courage: things are nowhere near as bad as they might seem. The modern treatment of diabetes is so successful that virtually every child who has it will nonetheless grow up to be a pretty healthy adult.

However, as diabetes isn't normally a curable condition, both parents and child have to realise that if a youngster is to avoid becoming seriously ill, he must stick to his treatment throughout his entire life. The most important parts of the treatment are diet and insulin injections.

The diet and the type of insulin, the quantity and the precise time at which it should be given are all prescribed by the specialist.

Young diabetic children very rapidly learn how to measure out their dose of insulin in the syringe and give themselves the jab. In many ways, they are a lot braver than we are.

DIARRHOEA *(See **Bowel Problems**)*

DOWN'S SYNDROME
Down's syndrome is an extraordinarily common form of mental handicap, occurring about once in every 600 births.

The incidence is much greater in the babies of older mothers. In women over 35 years, the risk starts rising rapidly, reaching one in 50 if the expectant mother is aged 45. This is why older mothers are offered an amniocentesis test in early pregnancy. A screening test which can be done on a simple blood sample is gradually being introduced for mothers of all ages, but it does *not* pick up all cases.

DUST ALLERGY
Many children are allergic to dust – or (to be more accurate) to the tiny mites which so often live in house dust.

The symptoms which this allergy produces are really exactly the same as those of hay fever *(see **Hay Fever**),* for example sneezing, runny nose and red, watery eyes.

Dust-mite allergy can't actually be cured but it can be controlled by the same sort of medications which are used for hay fever – nasal sprays such as Beconase and Rynacrom, and antihistamine pills. Naturally, you should also make every effort to reduce the amount of dust with which the child comes into contact.

Removal of dust-attracting furnishings may help, as well as a careful vacuum of the bedroom; enclose mattresses and pillows in covers that are specially designed to prevent the mites coming into contact with humans. These are available from some chemists' shops.

DYSLEXIA
A profound difficulty in reading (and writing), thought to be caused by a localised problem in the area of the brain which deals with perception of the written word.

It is important to realise that if your child is dyslexic, this does not mean that she is stupid. Many clever and gifted people have the disorder. With special help, dyslexic children can achieve excellent school results.

EAR ACHE
Ear ache (otitis media) is an inflammation of the middle ear. This is the little cavity which lies behind the ear drum, and which contains the tiny bones that transmit the sounds we hear from the drum to the inner ear.

The inflammation is caused by germs, which don't get in through the ear itself, but actually come up from the throat.

The middle ear cavity is connected to the throat by a narrow canal called the Eustachian tube. When a child has a sore throat or a cold, it is very easy for germs to find their way up this tube and into the ear. Once established there, they may cause inflammation and generate pus, thus producing pain. That's why so many children have ear ache after a cold.

Of course, a four-or five-year-old can tell you where the pain is; but if your child is too young to talk, you may well have considerable difficulty in making out what's wrong with him. A baby with ear ache may hold his ear or keep rubbing it, but he may just scream, and keep screaming

What should alert you to the possibility of ear ache is the baby's temperature. If it remains over 37.8°C (100°F) for several hours, and if he keeps screaming, then it is very likely that he has more than just an ordinary cold, and you should make sure his ears are checked by your family doctor. In the meantime, the child must have adequate relief for his pain.

One simple pain-relieving measure is to place a hot water bottle wrapped in a cloth over a child's ear. With a baby or a very young toddler you mustn't do this in case you burn him. It may be better to use a hot pad, for instance a towel that has been heated on the radiator and which you replace with another every few minutes as the first one cools down.

Second, give the child paracetamol, taking care not to exceed the stated dose for his age.

Your GP may come and see the child or he may ask for him to be brought to the surgery.

When the doctor sees your youngster, he'll inspect the child's ear drum with an instrument called an auriscope – and if he confirms that the condition is present, he will probably prescribe antibiotics for him.

Slight deafness during an attack of otitis media is common. However some children's hearing is permanently affected afterwards, so it is a good idea to make a rough check a month or so after the attack. If your child has trouble hearing a whisper across a room, or a watch held close to his ear, ask your doctor to see him again and if necessary arrange for the child to have a full hearing test (see **Deafness**).

EATING DISORDERS

This term mainly covers the well-known conditions called anorexia nervosa (in which the sufferer eats very little) and bulimia (in which she goes in for extreme bouts of over-eating).

Fortunately, neither is common in young children. But they are increasingly frequently encountered in the early adolescent years.

The precise cause of these disorders is not known, but they do often seem to be linked with stresses inside the family, and perhaps also with battles about feeding in early life. (Clearly, such confrontations should be avoided).

Treatment of eating disorders is very difficult, but if you suspect that your child is developing one, please go and talk over the matter with your GP. In a number of countries there are now self-help

organisations for patients with eating disorders;
their advice can be invaluable to the whole family.

ECZEMA

Vast numbers of children have eczema. Sadly,
many of them go through a lot of unnecessary
misery because people are unpleasant to them
on account of the appearance of their skin.
Eczema is not an infection. Regrettably, many
people see a patch of eczematous skin and think
that it must be infectious. That's why a child with
bad eczema may sometimes have a difficult time
at school from unthinking classmates.

Eczema is an inflammation of the skin, which is
often caused by an allergy and is more common
in children who have been bottle-fed than children
who have been breast-fed. The inflammation
produces itchy red patches on the skin - often
with uncomfortable cracks and a certain amount
of oozing of fluid from the affected areas.

During babyhood eczema often starts at around
the age of three months or so, and may come as
a nasty shock to the mother - particularly if she's
terribly proud of her new born and very upset by
the idea of other people seeing a flaw in his
appearance.

But if the patches of eczema aren't very extensive, there really is no cause for alarm. Small
patches don't usually distress the child; he's
blissfully unaware of them. So it is important to
try and maintain a detached attitude if possible.

In a few cases, it is possible to identify an underlying factor which is causing the inflammation.
There are many treatments for childhood eczema,
including bland emollients, steroid applications,

and coal tar. Your GP, paediatrician or dermatologist will advise you what's best. In general, soap and warm water are *not* good for the affected areas of skin.

EPILEPSY

Epilepsy is common, and it causes a great deal of stress and grief for affected children (and their parents). Much of this is quite unnecessary and unfair, because it is caused by the prejudice of others.

There are quite a lot of different types of epilepsy; it's not just one disease but lots of different ones. The two best-known types of epilepsy are **petit mal** and **grand mal**.

In petit mal the child just stops what he is doing and stares blankly into space for a little while, completely oblivious of what's going on around him. In such cases, you don't need to do anything in the way of first aid – just wait until he recovers.

Grand mal is more of a problem to cope with. This is the kind of fit in which the child falls down unconscious, shakes all over and may wet himself. It's alarming for the watcher, particularly as the victim may look as though he's going to die. In reality, however, the child feels no pain or discomfort while the fit is going on. Recovery will normally take place within a couple of minutes. All you have to do is to place him on a soft comfortable surface where he can't injure himself, and turn him on his side. Loosen the clothing at his neck so that he can breathe easily as he comes round.

Don't try to jam anything between his teeth. The only other first aid measure you should remember is to take his temperature when he's recovered from the convulsion. If it's over about 38.6°C (101.5°F), strip his clothes off, sponge him down with tepid water, and give him some paracetamol to bring his temperature down *(see Feverish Convulsions)*.

Epilepsy is caused by an electrical storm in the brain; it's like an exaggeration of the sudden paroxysm of brain activity caused by sneezing. In most children with epilepsy we have no idea at all why this electrical storm should occur.

Treatment. Once the diagnosis has been made, the child will be started on anti-convulsant drugs. There are many kinds of drug available, and the paediatrician or neurologist (nerve specialist) will probably have to experiment for some time before she finds the right combination and dose to suit a particular child's needs.

Once a suitable drug has been found it is absolutely essential that the pills or capsules are taken every day, exactly as prescribed.

Among children who are taking medication on a regular basis, the results of treatment are very good. Between 80 and 90 per cent usually show a satisfactory degree of suppression of fits.Most parents find it is relatively easy to cope with a child who only has a few convulsions each year, although obviously it's necessary to have your child take care about such sporting activities as cycling, swimming and horse-riding.

FAINTING
Fainting isn't usually a sign of anything seriously wrong. Many healthy children – and adults – faint occasionally. However, if it happens more than

once, you should consult your doctor. Fainting may be a symptom of another problem.

A faint is caused by blood draining away from the brain towards the legs and feet. This is most likely to happen if a child has suddenly jumped up from a lying position, or if he is feeling under the weather. A child may also faint if it is very hot. Emotional stress can have the same effect.

Treatment is just simply to keep the child lying down until he has recovered. Resist any tendency of well-meaning bystanders to put him into a sitting or standing position.

FATNESS

Far too many children in Western countries are very overweight.Only very rarely is this caused by a glandular problem, as some fond parents claim. Ninety-nine times out of one hundred the trouble is that the child eats far too many calories. Another factor may be lack of exercise.

Some children eat too much because they're unhappy. Other children are simply given far too large quantities of food by their parents, who often set a bad example by eating far too much themselves.

So, if your child is too fat, set a good example by cutting down on the stodgy, fatty things which you buy or cook. Take him to your doctor and get a strict diet sheet. If necessary, ask for an appointment with the local hospital dietician.

But please don't try to pressurise your GP into putting your child on slimming pills; these are powerful, dangerous and unlikely to work.

FEVER *(see **Temperature** and **Feverish Convulsions**)*

FEVERISH CONVULSIONS

If your youngster has a convulsion or fit (as vast numbers of children do every year), your doctor will very likely tell you that she thinks it was just a feverish (or febrile) convulsion.

Most convulsions in childhood aren't caused by full-blown epilepsy *(see **Epilepsy**)*, but by the effect of a raised temperature on the brain. The young brain is very immature – and often unable to stand up to changes in temperature.

In many children the brain simply cannot cope with a body temperature of more than about 38.9°C (102°F). So if the child has a bad cold or tonsillitis, and develops such a temperature, the brain responds by producing a convulsion.

If your child has had just one feverish convulsion, your doctor may feel that it is unnecessary to subject him to a lot of investigation. But any child who's had more than one should definitely be investigated.

Your GP will refer the child to the local specialist, who will examine him and carry out some tests. This includes the test known as an EEG, which stands for 'electroencephalogram'. The EEG is an electrical test of brain activity.

In the light of the results he obtains, the doctor will advise you as to whether your child needs to take medication every day in order to try to keep further fits away.

For very understandable reasons, parents tend to make one serious error in looking after children with temperatures. When their youngsters are ill, they do tend to keep the patient too warm

So if your child has already shown a tendency to feverish convulsions, then you will have to be prepared to bring his temperature *down* whenever he's feverish.

At the first sign of any feverishness, check his temperature every few hours. If it's above 38.3°C (101°F) taken by mouth, then he must be cooled down until his temperature is well below danger levels. Give him a a small amount of paracetamol, and remove any thick blankets or eiderdowns and woolly underwear.

If you just let him lie under a sheet, in a bedroom that is kept reasonably cool, this will probably be enough to lower his temperature.

If his thermometer reading is still the same after half an hour or so, however, then you should immediately carry out the procedure known as tepid sponging.

 This just means spending a few minutes wiping his limbs and body down with coolish water. It may also be helpful to play an electric fan on him, if you have one.

These measures will cool most children who have a tendency to convulsions, and take them out of the danger area on the thermometer. Do not be swayed by relatives' opinions: by cooling your child down, you are doing the very best possible thing and *not* giving him pneumonia.

FIBROCYSTIC DISEASE *(See Cystic Fibrosis)*

FIFTH DISEASE *(Erythema infectiosum)*

This is a very common infection of childhood, although its name is virtually unknown to parents and the general public.

The disease is given the name 'fifth disease' because it was discovered after scientists had identified four other common causes of fever and rash in childhood (German measles, measles, roseola and chickenpox).

It has recently been shown that fifth disease is almost certainly caused by a virus. The period of incubation is seven to fourteen days, after which the child may develop a slight temperature and perhaps a sore throat.

But what is really striking is the rash. This looks exactly as if the child has been slapped across the face - hence the alternative name 'Slapped Cheek Syndrome'. A rash may develop on the arms, legs and bottom. But the condition is not serious, and will soon clear up.

FITS *(see Epilepsy and Feverish Convulsions)*

FLAT FEET

This condition is one in which the arches (curves) under the child's feet simply aren't high enough. It can cause some pain in the calves.

The cause of flat feet isn't known. Fortunately, the condition doesn't matter all that much. An orthopaedic surgeon will tell you whether any treatment is really desirable or not. The possible therapies include foot exercises, supports in the shoes and surgery.

'FLU *(see **Influenza**)*

FOOD POISONING
This is caused by germs contaminating food.

Symptoms of food poisoning include tummy ache, diarrhoea and vomiting. If you suspect a case of food poisoning in your family, put the victims to bed, call a doctor, and if possible save the food so that tests can be done on it.

Food poisoning is alarmingly common in many Western countries, partly because much of the frozen poultry you buy in shops is contaminated with salmonella germs. To try and prevent food poisoning, follow these strict rules:

1 Don't put poultry or meat that is defrosting in places where it can drip onto other foods

2 Don't put it on working surfaces which you are then going to use for other foods unless you have thoroughly scrubbed the surface first

3 Defrost frozen poultry and meat thoroughly

4 Cook it thoroughly too

5 Don't let anyone with an infected finger or hand prepare food

6 Make sure all food-handlers in your home wash their hands after going to the loo

7 Don't leave warm meat dishes around (particularly uncovered ones) to cool slowly, with a view to reheating them later. Put them in the fridge, or cook only small portions, as these will cool faster

FRACTURES

'Fracture' means exactly the same as 'break'.
Broken bones are common in childhood, more so
in boys than in girls. Fortunately, most fractures
are simply very painful, rather than very serious
and dangerous.

If you suspect a broken bone:

* Immobilise the affected bit of your child by
  gently splinting it to something firm (e.g. a
  walking stick)
* Take him to the nearest accident and
  emergency department, since an X-ray will
  nearly always be needed
* Don't give him any food or drink

If the X-ray shows that the fracture hasn't caused
any deformity of the bone, the doctor may put on
a plaster of Paris (or similar arrangement that
immobilises the limb) to keep the bone-ends
steady until they knit together.

If the fracture has caused a deformity of the
bone, then the doctor will have to reduce it. This
just means putting the bone straight, and it has
to be done under a general anaesthetic. This is
why you should not give any food or drink to a
child who has a possible fracture.

GAS POISONING

Gas poisoning most commonly occurs in flats
(particularly holiday flats), caravans, boats and
other enclosed living quarters which have badly
ventilated heaters. Victims of gas poisoning are
found unconscious, and often bright pink.

Immediate action: drag the child into clean air
quickly (before you yourself are overcome). Give

the kiss of life. If his heart has stopped, give heart massage. Call an ambulance!

GASTROENTERITIS
(see **Food Poisoning,** and **Bowel Problems**)

GERMAN MEASLES (Rubella)
This is a mild infection for a child, but possibly a very serious one for an expectant mother.

Children catch the rubella virus from other people who have it; the virus is sprayed into the air as an infected child or adult breathes, sneezes, laughs or talks. It then enters somebody else's nose or mouth. About 14 to 20 days later, the youngster will probably get German measles.

The symptoms of German measles vary wildly; an affected child may well not have any obvious symptoms at all. She may not even have a rash. But many children with German measles do have a rash – a bumpy brownish-pink one that usually spreads over the body.

At the same time, the child may become slightly off-colour, possibly with a mild sore throat. A good clue is that the glands at the back of his neck are usually enlarged.

Your doctor should see the child to confirm the diagnosis - but please don't take her down to the surgery, where there might be expectant mothers in the waiting rooms.

No treatment is needed, but your doctor will doubtless advise keeping her at home for at least a few days, for fear of infecting pregnant women she may come into contact with.

Immunization schedules against rubella vary from country to country. But whenever it's available, do have your child immunized.

GLANDULAR FEVER (Infectious Mononucleosis)

This is a virus infection that is common in teenagers, and also occurs in younger children.

The virus is believed to be spread from mouth to mouth by talking, laughing, sneezing, coughing and perhaps kissing.

Infectious mononucleosis is thought to come on about one-and-a-half weeks after exposure. The symptoms are tiredness and weakness, fever, sore throat and swollen glands. The doctor will confirm the diagnosis by taking a blood sample.

GRAZES

Grazes are jolly painful for the child, and every parent knows the experience of having a toddler scream the place down after having the skin scraped off his knees.

However, these painful but minor skin grazes will never give any serious trouble as long as you wash the child's skin carefully with soap and warm water, and take care to get rid of any gravel or any dirt.

Any of the standard proprietary antiseptics which you can purchase from your local chemist can then be applied.

If the graze is extensive, dress it with an adhesive plaster. Or if it's very big, cover it with a square of sterile gauze.

GUM PROBLEMS

Gum disorders are not very common in children, provided they clean their teeth twice daily and see their dentist twice a year.

But bleeding gums may indicate a problem, and should be checked out by a dentist without delay. Large, painful lumps on the gum are usually abscesses caused by infection from decayed teeth: the child should see a dentist as soon as possible so that the abscess can be dealt with.

HARE LIP *(see **Cleft Palate** and **Hare Lip**)*

HAY FEVER

In hay fever, the child develops running eyes and starts sneezing and snuffling in the grass-pollen season which in Northern Europe will arrive in April or May, depending on the weather.

In other countries, hay fever arrives at other times; in the United States, it mainly happens during the ragweed pollen season, in the autumn.

The diagnosis is usually obvious although some children are wrongly thought to have recurrent colds, not hay fever. Treatment has improved recently; the main types are as follows:

* Older forms of anti-histamine pills and medicine. These have the disadvantage of making many children sleepy;

* Newer anti-histamines, which have no real sedative effect

* Steroid inhalers, which are very useful, but do not sedate

* Nasal anti-allergy drugs. Versions of these can be used in the child's eyes, to combat the disabling wateriness and redness. Note that these drugs must be used long-term for their protective effect – it's no good trying to use them to treat a sudden attack of hay fever.

De-sensitizing injections are now less used than they once were, because there is always the risk of a serious reaction to the jabs. However, don't forget the following commonsense ways of combatting hay fever:

* If possible, keep your windows closed on warm, dry days, when the pollen count is likely to be high

* Keep car windows closed

* Consider wrap-around sunglasses to keep the pollen out of your child's eyes

* Also consider trying an 'anti-smog' mask over the mouth and nose

* If all else fails, taking the child to the seaside (or anywhere else where pollen counts are low) may help

HEADACHE
Headache isn't usually serious, except in rare cases *(see **Meningitis**)*. Possible causes include:

* Any feverish illnesses (colds, 'flu, etc.)

* Sinusitis *(see **Sinusitis**)*

* Stress

* Head injury

* Migraine *(see **Migraine**)*.

Eye strain is often said by adults to be the cause of headache, but this seems a bit doubtful. However, if your child has recurrent headaches, it certainly does no harm to have his eyes checked by an optician.

HEART DISORDERS
These are now rare among children in most Western countries, but congenital abnormalities of the heart do occur in babies, usually for no known reason. The more common abnormalities are holes in the heart and malpositioning of the tubes leading into or out of the heart. Fortunately, many of these abnormalities can now be corrected by surgery – even possibly by heart transplantation in a few cases.

Cardiomyopathy is a term used to indicate one of a group of disorders in which there is a serious abnormality of the muscle which makes up the heart. In childhood cases, the cause is virtually always unknown. Treatment is with drugs to help the ailing heart muscle to pump. In a few cases a heart transplant is a possibility.

Rheumatic heart disease (caused by rheumatic fever) affects the heart valves; in Western countries it has become very rare during the last few decades.

HEPATITIS
This means 'inflammation of the liver'. There are various types; for the commonest variety in Western countries *see **Jaundice**.*

HERNIA

This is the same thing as a rupture. In other words, it's a condition where part of a child's internal organs start bulging through a weak spot, for example in the abdominal wall. The most common such weak spots occur in (a) the groin; (b) the navel.

Groin hernias These are quite common in young children, especially boys. The symptom is a bulge near the junction of the inner thigh and trunk.

Navel (umbilical) hernias The navel tends to be a weak place, and young babies frequently have a mild hernia there. For some reason, these little ruptures are specially common in babies of Afro-Caribbean extraction.

Fortunately, very small navel bulges will often go away as the child's tummy muscles get stronger. Apart from this, all hernias need to be treated with a simple operation.

HICCUPS (HICCOUGHS)

Most cases of hiccups stop by themselves. Where this doesn't happen, it is worth trying a traditional remedy such as drinking out of the wrong side of a glass or putting a tiny spot of salt on the child's tongue (but only if she agrees).

HIP PROBLEMS (see Congenital Dislocation of the Hip)

HODGKIN'S DISEASE

This serious disorder of the lymph glands affects some young adults and older children. The cause isn't known. Symptoms include painless swelling of the glands in the neck, armpits and groin; weakness; and sometimes jaundice.

These days, the outlook is good for Hodgkin's disease, and most children who get it can now be cured – although the cure will take some years. Treatment is with powerful anti-cancer type drugs and radiotherapy.

HYDROCEPHALUS

This means 'water on the brain'. It is a serious condition, mostly occurring in the first year of life. The classic symptom is marked enlargement of the child's skull. This is caused by a blockage of the drainage tube through which brain fluid (CSF) normally drains away.

Hydrocephalus is not easy to treat, but this position was improved many years ago when an American engineer whose own child was dying of hydrocephalus sat down and designed a brilliantly simple valve which could be implanted into the child's body by a surgeon – and which would drain off the excess fluid.

With the aid of this device and its successors (and also with drug treatment) the lives of many babies with hydrocephalus have been saved.

HYPERACTIVITY

Hyperactivity just means having too much activity or energy. All children are far too active at times, and can try their parents' patience and wear them to a frazzle as a result.

There are some children however whose level of activity is way above normal, and who constantly cause chaos and disruption. In some cases this behaviour is caused by brain damage, and in some it is the result of serious psychological problems, which are often linked with problems in the family.

In recent years, there have been attempts to link food additives (particularly the common yellow dye called 'tartrazine') to hyperactivity. On the whole, doctors have been less than enthusiastic about some of the claims which have been made. But it is possible that your local hyperactivity self-help group can help you to identify a food item which may be causing your child problems, and which you can try removing from his diet.

HYSTERIA

This is a state – common in older children (girls more than boys) – in which the child produces symptoms which have no physical cause. In other words, the symptom – which is quite frequently dramatic and sometimes bizarre – is due to some emotional causes.

This doesn't mean the youngster is making it up or pretending; she isn't. In most cases, she believes fervently in the genuineness of her symptoms, and may be frightened by them. Some of the most common hysterical symptoms include a sudden collapse, inexplicable blindness, an inability to speak, paralysis and also a loss of consciousness.

In some cases, an important factor may be over-breathing (hyperventilation). It is not generally realised that if a child (or adult) gets a bit het up and starts breathing too fast, this rapid breathing may have a disorientating effect on the brain – because it 'washes out' too much carbon dioxide from the body.

For this reason, the simple procedure of getting an over-excited, hysterical child to breathe into a paper bag may be sucessful. Breathing into the paper bag builds up the body's carbon dioxide again. The results can be dramatic.

IMMUNIZATIONS

Every child should have the protection of all the available immunizations unless there is some good reason why not; in other words if there is some real contra-indication.

Unfortunately, a very substantial minority of children miss out on some or all of the available vaccinations – sometimes because their parents have fears about one particular jab.

Remember that if you feel strongly opposed to an individual immunization, you can always let your child have all the rest.

Immunization schedules vary greatly from country to country, but in most Western nations children are offered the following:

* Polio, given by drops

* Diphtheria, lockjaw (tetanus), whooping cough, measles, mumps, German measles (rubella), Hib (haemophilus), all administered by injection.

In addition, protection against tuberculosis (TB) by BCG immunization is offered in the majority of countries.

In hotter parts of the world it may be necessary to immunize against such diseases as typhoid and yellow fever.

IMPETIGO

This childhood skin infection is usually caused by the staphylococcus germ – the one which you find in boils and styes. This causes a golden, crusty blistery eruption on the child's skin – most often on his face, although it can appear in other places. It is spread by direct contact.

Impetigo isn't serious, and these days is quickly cleared up with antibiotic cream (and possibly some form of medicine).

INFLUENZA

'Flu isn't usually a life-threatening illness in a child although it can make your child feel extremely miserable.

So It is important to get medical help, because there is a small risk of complications such as pneumonia or ear ache.

'Flu is caused by a virus, and influenza viruses go around the world in quite dramatic outbreaks. So usually, the newspapers or TV news will have alerted you to the fact that there's a lot of 'flu around.

Symptoms of 'flu may include cold symptoms such as sneezing, severe aches and pains all over, a high temperature, weakness and, in a minority of cases, diarrhoea or vomiting.

If you suspect 'flu, keep the child at home (don't go down to the surgery) and phone the doctor.

She will probably suggest paracetamol, and advise plenty of fluids and bed rest till the child feels well. Usually the illness will be over in about four days – so contact the doctor again if the child doesn't improve or if her condition takes a turn for the worse for no apparent reason. *DO NOT* give aspirin. *(See **Reye's Syndrome**)*.

INTUSSUSCEPTION

This is a 'telescoping' of the child's bowel – in other words, one part slides inside the next bit. It produces a severe tummy ache and often rectal bleeding, as well as blockage of the bowels.

Intussusception is most common round about the time a baby is weaned; it may be that when solid food is introduced this sparks it off.

In the old days, intussusception could be fatal, but today prompt intervention by a surgeon will cure the problem.

JAUNDICE

This is a yellowness of the child's skin and eyes, caused by a build-up of yellow bile pigment. There are literally dozens of possible causes of jaundice in childhood. Fortunately, the outlook in most cases is good. The following is a list of the more common causes.

In the newborn:
* Jaundice of prematurity is common in premature babies. Usually fades in days.

* Jaundice caused by Rhesus factor: Increasingly rare today, as vulnerable women often have a protective injection.

Toddlers and schoolchildren:
* Infectious hepatitis (infective jaundice). The cause is a virus which affects the liver. The child usually becomes ill about six weeks

after she has been exposed to the virus, although there are some types which have a much longer period of incubation. The main treatment is bed rest.

* Nearly all children recover completely in about a month's time, although a very small proportion develop more serious liver disease.

LEUKAEMIA

Leukaemia is one of the most frightening of the childhood illnesses, and many parents dread the possibility of this disorder striking their child.

However, the outlook is nowhere as bleak as it used to be a few years ago, and if a child gets leukaemia (particularly what is called the 'acute lymphatic' form) there is now a very good chance that he can be cured.

Leukaemia is a cancer of the white blood cells. Blood contains two main types of cell: red cells and white cells.

White cells are concerned with important jobs such as mopping up germs that try to get into the body, and helping to maintain the child's immunity to infections.

These white cells are manufactured mainly in the bone marrow – which can be found inside many bones in our body.

White cells are 'turned out' all the time, and in very great numbers, and the reason for this is that they are constantly being worn out by the various defensive functions they have to perrorm around the body.

What happens in leukaemia is that white cells start being produced in very large numbers. This over-production of cells is typical of cancers.

In fact, that's what cancer really means: a sudden loss of control over the cells in some part of the body, so that they reproduce at frightening speed, producing masses of destructive cells.

The leukaemic child's blood is full of white cells – and, unfortunately, these are very immature white cells which are no good at protecting the child against the germs to which he is exposed every day of his life.

As a result, within a very short time the child has virtually no defence against infection. At the same time, the surfeit of abnormal white cells in his body makes him weak and run-down. There is usually an associated anaemia; that is, a lack of red cells so that he may look pale and wan.

The main features of leukaemia tend to include paleness, weakness, anaemia that does not respond to treatment, enlargement of the spleen, and recurrent unexplained bleeding.

The diagnosis is made by taking a blood test.

Once the disease has been diagnosed, treatment is with anti-cancer drugs, radiation and (where possible) a bone marrow transplant.

LICE

There are various types of lice which affect humans, but in Western countries there is one common type which affects children – the head louse. This particular louse causes an intense itching of the scalp.

To many parents this is an embarrassing subject and they are very reluctant even to admit the possibility that their youngster might have nits (as head lice are often called).

But your child can't help getting them – and there's no way you can prevent him from catching them.

While on your child's head, the louse takes an occasional bite out of the scalp and, from time to time, lays little white eggs which stick to the base of the hair.

Since all children touch heads with each other at school – dozens of times a day, in fact – it's easy for the louse to leap from one child's head to another, childs head.

Indeed they can jump from your childs head onto yours. So when your youngster does get nits, the whole family must be thoroughly treated.

Special preparations are used to treat live. Your doctor will advise you about them.

LOCKJAW (Tetanus)

This very serious infection is caused by germs which are found in soil, gravel and also on road surfaces. The germs get into cuts (particularly deep ones) and produce a special chemical which paralyses the muscles, and may be fatal.

Tetanus is now fairly rare in most countries in the west, because of the very effective immunization which is used to prevent it.

But if your child sustains a deep or dirty cut – particularly one contaminated by soil – always wash it very carefully and then take him to an accident department or to a doctor.

MEASLES

In countries where vaccination is routine, this infection is fortunately much rarer than it was. Warning: it can have very nasty complications. Although many parents still think of measles as a trivial disorder, in fact it can kill.

Measles has an incubation period of about 10 days at the end of which the child gets cold-like symptoms and runny eyes. Four days later, she gets a rash which starts behind the ears and spreads across the body.

In uncomplicated cases, the youngster will get better of her own accord in about a week. But some children develop serious complications affecting the brain, ear and chest, so it's well worth getting your child immunized.

MENINGITIS

This very serious infection of the membranes which cover the child's brain is caused by one of various types of germ, usually breathed in from a person who is a healthy carrier of it.

Fortunately, meningitis is quite rare in most Western countries.

Regrettably, the very rareness of meningitis makes it quite difficult for doctors to diagnose. So the danger of meningitis is that it may go unrecognised until it is too late.

Symptoms to look out for are: severe headache, stiffness of the neck, dislike of the light, raised temperature, confusion and, sometimes, a purple or reddish rash.

If you ever suspect meningitis in your child, ring your doctor **immediately** and tell her why you're worried. If after examination thje doctor thinks that meningitis is a possibility, she'll admit the child to hospital.

At the hospital a doctor will carry out a test called a lumbar puncture. This involves tapping off some fluid from the spine.

The test makes clear whether the child has meningitis, and indicates exactly which germs are responsible – and which antibioticwill be most effective in destroying them.

If the course of antibiotics is started promptly, there's an excellent chance of the child's swift and complete recovery. The recently introduced Hib vaccine protects children against one type of meningitis.

MIGRAINE

This common condition is believed to be caused by an odd reaction in the arteries (blood-carrying tubes) inside the skull.

The most usual symptom is severe headache, which is usually felt only on one side of the head. The headache is often preceded by odd visual disturbances – for instance, a sensation of seeing dazzling lights or zig-zag lines.

Soon after the attack, the child often vomits. Naturally, this causes an extra problem, in that any anti-migraine tablet given to him may well not be absorbed into the system.

It's not clear why some children should get migraine, while others don't. There seems to be a marked family tendency, so probably there is a hereditary factor which makes the arteries in the skull react in this odd way to certain provoking factors.

Stress – including exam stress – may be one such factor. Chocolate and oranges have been known for many years to trigger off migraine attacks in some people.

When your child gets an attack of migraine, take the following steps. Lie him down in a darkened room and give him paracetamol as soon you can (before the migraine upsets his stomach and interferes with the absorption of the pills).

If your doctor has suggested a 'stomach-settling' drug, such as metoclopramide, give it as early as you can in the attack; with luck, this will ensure that the paracetamol is absorbed.

Remember to put a bucket or bowl by the bed, in case he's sick, and **let him** go to sleep if he wants to. In most cases, he will feel much better after a brief doze

MONONUCLEOSIS (see *Glandular Fever*)

MUMPS (Parotitis)
This infection is now much rarer than it used to be in countries where mumps vaccine is widely used. The incubation period is about 18-28 days. At the end of this time the child becomes generally unwell, and then one or both cheeks start to swell up. This is due to inflammation of the two big saliva glands (the parotids) which lie on either

side of the mouth. The swellings are very painful, especially when eating.

Mumps don't respond to antibiotics, so all that a doctor can advise is to put the child to bed with lots of cool drinks and some pain-killers. **DO NOT give aspirin**.

With luck he will recover in about 10 days or so. But occasionally children get painful inflammation of the testicles or the ovaries, or (rarely) brain inflammation. So the mumps vaccine is definitely worth having.

NAPPY RASH

Nappy rash can be pretty distressing – for parents as well as the child. But it will always get better eventually.

Very often the best treatment for nappy rash is to expose the child's bottom. Certainly, in all cases, you should stop using plastic pants until the child is completely better. This is a difficult point for doctors to get over to many parents. This is understandable, of course, because it's Mum (and not the doctor) who has to clear up the mess caused by a baby who is not wearing a pair of plastic pants.

In most cases, nappy rash occurs because the urine in the baby's wet nappy is in contact with the child's skin for too long. Germs break down chemicals in this urine to form ammonia – a strong irritant to the baby's skin.

Since the ammonia can't evaporate (because of the plastic pants), it attacks the poor old baby's bottom – causing a red and/or spotty rash. If you notice that a nappy rash is appearing, stop using plastic pants and whenever possible, let the child go without nappies, so that the sun and air get to her bottom.

After any soiling wash baby's bottom thoroughly, dry it gently, and then apply a barrier cream.

If these measures don't work, you'll have to seek expert professional help from your doctor or health visitor.

NERVOUS STRESS

Quite understandably many children do suffer from nervous stress – and this usually causes physical symptoms.

The symptoms which are often produced as a reaction to emotional distress seem to be very genuine to them. Common symptoms are: tummy ache, headache, feeling sick, feeling faint, having to rush to the loos, constipation, burping, tics and nightmares.

Some children also develop irrational fears, a compulsion to keep counting and checking things, or a violent aversion to going to school.

So what are the stresses which can provoke these symptoms in children? Again and again, they fall into one of two categories.

Trouble at school may involve being bullied, or being frightened of a particular teacher, or being irrationally upset about not being able to keep up with work.

Trouble at home usually seems to be related to divorce or to other marriage difficulties between the parents. Unfortunately, these days we are increasingly aware that some children are under a lot of stress because of brutality, or even because of sexual abuse.

If you suspect your child is suffering from stress then don't try to solve the problem by having him put on tranquillisers. The important thing is to try to get to the bottom of whatever is causing the stress. Your GP should be able to help you, and she may well suggest that family therapy would be a good idea.

NIGHTMARES

Nearly all children get nightmares at some time, and they can be very frightening. The factors which can provoke them include:

* Worry and emotional stress (see **Nervous Stress**)

* Seeing frightening films or TV programmes

* A feverish illness

If your child just has an occasional nightmare, then there's no need to worry. When she wakes up frightened, or stumbles terrified into your room in the middle of the night, just give her a cuddle and explain to her that everything is all right.

But if nightmares are really persistent and they are causing a lot of distress, you need to do something about it. Begin by asking yourself whether it's caused by any trouble at home or at school. (Is it, for instance, just the arrival of a new baby which has unsettled your child?)

If this commonsense measure fails, then talk things over with your doctor. If she can't diagnose the problem, then it may be necessary to consult a psychologist or other qualified counsellor.

NOSEBLEEDS

To treat a nosebleed:

1   Sit the child up

2   Squeeze the soft part of her nose firmly between finger and thumb. Keep the pressure up for at least ten minutes. Resist the temptation to relax the pressure and 'peek'. This is the most common reason for failure of the treatment

3   Don't push cotton wool or anything else into the nostrils

4   When the child has recovered, don't let her blow her nose for at least three hours

In very rare cases, bleeding is uncontrollable by these means, and you'll have to take the child to an Accident and Emergency department.

P.K.U. *(see **Phenylketonuria**)*

PARACETAMOL

This is a very useful drug for relieving pain and lowering a raised temperature. In recent years parents have been choosing paracetamol instead of aspirin because of there is the risk that aspirin can cause the illness known as Reye's syndrome *(see **Reye's Syndrome**)*. Paracetamol is about as effective as aspirin as a pain-killer, and is also useful in childhood fevers but it doesnt have the anti-inflammatiory effect that aspirin has.

Paracetamol does not cause the major side-effect of aspirin – irritation of the stomach – and it hasn't (so far, anyway) been linked in any way with Reye's syndrome.

The liquid preparations (sold under different brand names) are easy to give to children.

But please remember that paracetamol is a drug, even though people think of it as being very mild.

If, like many parents, you keep it in your home, bear in mind that fatal overdoses of paracetamol do occur in children.

The great danger is that your child may decide to help herself to some more of those nice tablets (or that nice syrup) and so kill herself. So keep paracetamol in a safe place.

PETIT MAL (see *Epilepsy*)

PHENYLKETONURIA (PKU)
This rare but very important inherited disorder is important because:

* If untreated, it causes mental subnormality

* It can be detected soon after birth by a screening test on the child's blood

* Once it has been picked up, then the child's diet will need adjusting to prevent the mental subnormality

There are now many happy children who have completely normal intelligence because the screening test detected their phenylketonuria.

In most Western countries PKU occurs in one in twenty thousand babies.

Although it is inherited, parents will have no idea if they are carrying the gene for phenylketonuria. It is only when both a woman and her partner are carrying the gene responsible, and have a child, that the disease may occur.

PLEURISY

Pleurisy (which is known in some countries as pleuritis) is an inflammation of the membrane which surrounds the lungs.

Pleurisy can make the child very ill and can be distressing, mainly because it tends to cause intense pain in the chest area especially when the child takes deep breaths.

Pleurisy is usually secondary to some other chest problem, such as pneumonia *(see **Pneumonia**)*. The child needs to be admitted to hospital, but with antibiotic and other treatment should make a good recovery.

PNEUMONIA

This means inflammation of the lung. It's known in some countries as 'pneumonitis', and is nearly always caused by germs.

There are various kinds of pneumonia. Infants are most likely to contract bronchopneumonia while older children are more likely to contract lobar pneumonia.

Pneumonia used to be a very serious condition. But in this age of antibiotics, most children make a rapid recovery.

POISONING

For poisoning by gas *see* **Gas Poisoning**.

Treat any case of poisoning as potentially fatal. Never wait to see how things go just because the child seems quite well, or because you think he hasn't taken very much.

Always take the poison or the empty container to hospital with you; if the child has vomited, take a specimen of the vomited material as well.

If the child is unconscious, turn him on his side and remove anything (such as vomit) that is blocking the mouth. Make sure he can breathe, then **immediately phone for an ambulance**. Any delay in getting the child to hospital may be fatal.
.
If the substance he swallowed was a corrosive poison (such as an acid or alkali), or a petroleum product, he will probably scream with pain from his burned lips and mouth. Splash water across the burned areas and try to give him water or milk to drink.

If the child is conscious get him to hospital immediately.

POLIO

This word is short for 'poliomyelitis', which is a very serious virus infection that used to kill or paralyse many children.

Today it has almost disappeared in the West, thanks to polio immunization. However it may become more common again in the near future if parents don't make the responsible decision to have all their children immunized. (*See also* **Immunizations**)

PYLORIC STENOSIS

This is a narrowing of the tube which carries food out of the baby's stomach.

This moderately common disorder of young babies (aged one to twelve weeks) affects more boys than girls.

What happens is that the muscle round the tube leading out of the stomach becomes swollen, and the swelling 'comes up' whenever the child has a feed. We don't know why this swelling should occur, but the great thing is that it's easily cured these days.

The main symptom is forceful vomiting – what is called projectile vomiting. This means that your baby is so violently sick that the vomit may quite literally hit the wall on the other side of the room.

Once the diagnosis has been made, a surgeon can operate to relieve the obstruction. The child should make a good recovery.

REYE'S SYNDROME

Reye's syndrome (it rhymes with 'eyes') has been in the headlines for some time because there is a suggested link between aspirin products and this syndrome. As a result, children under the age of 12 are no longer given aspirin.

There has also been a suggestion that drugs that are administered to prevent vomiting might also be implicated.

Reye's syndrome is a very serious disease of the brain and liver. It attacks children recovering from some relatively minor illness – especially 'flu or chickenpox.

In some cases (not all), it seems likely that the syndrome is in some way triggered off by aspirin.

The death rate in Reye's syndrome is high, so clearly every parent ought to know the symptoms:

* In most cases, just as a child starts getting better after some relatively minor infection, she suddenly starts vomiting and the vomiting is severe and repeated

Other possible symptoms are:

* Deliriousness

* Fits and spasms of the arms or legs

* Staring into space

* Lethargy

* Screaming attacks

* Unconsciousness

If you are in any doubt at all call your doctor immediately for advice

RHEUMATOID ARTHRITIS
Unfortunately, this disabling condition occurs in children as well as adults.

Girls are affected three times as often as boys. Symptoms include persistent and very distressing pains in the joints,plus swelling and stiffness, especially in the hands.

Treatment is mainly with anti-inflammatory drugs plus physiotherapy. For severe cases joint replacement is often possible. Things often improve as the child gets older.

RINGWORM

Ringworm is a common skin infection, especially in country districts where a child may easily catch the disese through frequent contact with a wide variety of animals.

Ringworm is a fungus infection, and it produces an itchy, red crusty area on the child's skin. Very often the affected area has the curved edge that gives this infection its name. When it affects the scalp, it often causes a patch of hair loss.

Most children can be successfully treated with an anti-fungus cream or ointment. This must be prescribed by your doctor.

ROSEOLA INFANTUM

Although the name isn't known to the majority of parents, *Roseola infantum* is one of the common feverish rashes of childhood.

Its alternative name is *Exanthem subitum*. It most often occurs between the ages of six months and two years. Medical proffesionals are almost certain that this condition is the result of a virus.

The incubation period is 7-17 days; then the child develops a temperature lasting a few days. When the temperature falls, a rash develops.

The doctor will probably advise giving paracetamol tablets and keeping the patient cool. ***Don't give aspirin*** *(see **Reye's Syndrome**)*.The majority of children recover very quickly.

RUBELLA *(see **German Measles** and **Immunizations**)*

SCARLET FEVER *(Scarlatina)*

This used to be a serious condition which killed many children. But in most Western countries it is at present a mild infection, characterised by a sore throat and a rash.

Scarlet fever is caused by a common throat germ, the streptococcus. The incubation period is usually two or three days, after which the child develops a red throat, vomiting, a headache and a temperature. Within two days, the child will develop a rash over her body and face, but the area around her mouth will be spared.

Treatment is with penicillin and paracetamol. As kidney and heart complications occasionally occur, the doctor will want to test her urine and check her heart.

SICKLE CELL DISEASE

Rare in Western countries, this is a form of anaemia (weakness of the blood) which occurs in a small proportion of children who are of Afro-Caribbean ancestry.

The disease is caused by a gene that is carried by some 10 per cent of Afro-Caribbeans. In most cases, carrying this faulty gene causes very few problems at all, and the carriers are seldom aware that they have it. Problems arise when a woman and her partner are carriers and they have a child. In such cases there is a one in four chance that the child will have sickle cell anaemia. Statisticians have demonstrated that this is – fortunately– a rare occurrence. Of course it is always a tragedy for the parents and their child when it does occur.

This is because the features of sickle cell anaemia are severe growth stunting, weakness, tiredness, debility, jaundice and bouts of intense pains in the limbs.

It is best to get the child treated by a specialist who knows how to handle the severe, painful crisis of sickle cell anaemia. Many children now grow up to lead active lives.

SLEEP PROBLEMS

Unfortunately quite a lot of children do not sleep as long as their parents would wish – particularly in babyhood. And with babies it is very important to realise that there is no fixed number of hours that a child must sleep.

Babies vary greatly in the amount they need, and for some it is an entirely normal event to be awake and demanding the parents' attention at five in the morning.

The answer to babyhood wakefulness is not to give drugs. When the child wakes you, you should briefly satisfy her needs (for instance, feeding her or changing her) and then put her back to bed. If in doubt, ask your health visitor for advice.

Older children also vary enormously in the amount of sleep they need, and provided your family doctor says your child is healthy, you should not worry about how long she sleeps.

However, if a child suddenly starts lying awake for very long periods, this may very well be an indication of an emotional disturbance (for

instance, depression), and you should obtain
professional advice, beginning with your doctor.

SORE THROAT

A sore throat is usually caused by infection, but
irritation may play a part.

Oddly enough, most young children don't actually
complain of soreness in the throat. They usually
just feel unwell, and may cough or be sick. In
older children, a sore throat is exactly the same
as an adult's sore throat.

Most childhood sore throats are caused by a
virus: this means that no antibiotic in the world
will have any effect on them, as antibiotics only
work on bacteria.

A child with a sore throat should be kept at home
and given lots of fluid and a little paracetamol.
The proprietary throat lozenges, sweets and
sprays which you can buy cheaply from a chemist
are soothing although there's some doubt about
whether they really do much good.

If a child really feels terrible with a sore throat –
or if it goes on for some days – then contact your
doctor (*see* **Tonsilitis**).

SPRAINS

These are twists of a joint, with no fracture. Most
childhood sprains respond well to rest, to gentle
compressions with a bandage, and also to the
application of ice or a packet of frozen peas
wrapped in a towel.

If there is a lot of pain or distress, consult your
family doctor.

SQUINTS

A squint must never be ignored, so do not pay any attention to anybody who says 'Oh, don't worry, she'll grow out of it'. Beware also of those people who say 'Oh, it's just a lazy eye'. There really is no such thing as a lazy eye.

A genuine, persistent squint must be checked by an eye surgeon. This is necessary because an untreated squint can rapidly lead to permanent loss of vision in one eye.

STAMMERING (Stuttering)

Large numbers of children aged between two and six stammer a bit, simply because it's so difficult for an experienced young mouth to pour out all those complicated new words. Don't draw attention to your child if she does this: it's far better just to ignore it.

But if a child is clearly developing a bad stutter, then it's best to call in professional help as soon as possible. This means getting her to a speech therapist. With skilled speech therapy, many stammerers will be cured, and all should be very substantially improved.

STINGS

Bee Stings   In temperate countries, these are rarely serious. If the sting is still in the skin, remove it gently with a pair of tweezers or the blade of a knife. Don't squeeze the skin, as this may spread the poison.

In cases of multiple bee stings (which happens if a whole swarm of bees attacks somebody), stings in the mouth, or in the case of the child collapsing, get medical help as soon as possible.

Wasp Stings   These are usually fairly trivial and there is no actual sting to remove from the skin. However you should consult a doctor if the sting is in the mouth or if your child has a very bad reaction to it.

Cold compresses and paracetamol can be used to relieve pain. Pain-relief sprays available from chemists are useful.

If the child collapses, then you must get medical assistance immediately.

STOMACH PAIN *(See Tummy Ache)*

STYE
Styes are infections of the hair follicles from which the eyelashes grow. They are caused by the same infectious germs which are responsible for causing boils.

Bathe the child's eye with cotton wool dipped in warm water. If the stye fails to clear up in a few days – or if styes are recurrent – then you should consult your doctor.

SUNBURN
The best thing to do about sunburn is to prevent it, especially if your child is fair-skinned. Don't let him go out without a hat and a top on in the hot sun – particularly during the first day or two when you are on holiday.

Don't hesitate to apply plenty of a high-factor sun cream. If sunburn does occur in spite of your precautions, apply calamine lotion and, if necessary, give paracetamol for the pain.

SUNSTROKE

Symptoms include severe headache, weakness, irritability, thirst and even confusion. Amazingly, this kind of reaction among small children can occur after just a few hours' exposure to the sun in quite cool countries.

Treatment involves putting the youngster to bed in a darkened room, and giving him plenty of iced drinks. In those mild cases seen in temperate zones, he is usually better within 48 hours.

TAKING YOUR CHILD'S TEMPERATURE

You need a thermometer in the home, because children so often get raised temperatures.

The newer digital thermometers are very easy to use and to read, but most people still have the old mercury ones, on which yiou have to 'read off' the figure which the mercury n the central column reaches.

You can also buy fever strips from the chemist, which you apply to the child's forehead and then read off a reasonable approximation of the temperature.

To read a mercury thermometer, you may need a magnifying glass if you are long-sighted, but in practice most people are able to read the figures easily. Viewed from the side, the thermometer glass forms a type of lens, so that the column of mercury appears much wider than it really is, and so is easy to see.

In some countries, the figures are still in Fahrenheit degrees, but today the thermometers manufactured in most countries are tabulated in degrees Centigrade (degrees Celsius).

THERMOMETER READINGS

Fahrenheit	Centigrade	
95 96	35.0 35.6	Rather cold
97 98 99	36.1 36.7 37.2	Of no significance
100 101	37.8 38.3	Fairly warm – consult a doctor, especially if there are other symptoms.
102 103 104	38.9 39.4 40.0	VERY HOT – YOU **MUST** COOL THE CHILD DOWN AND RING THE DOCTOR
105 106	40.6 41.1	VERY, **VERY** HOT – GET **URGENT** MEDICAL HELP

Your thermometer will be marked in degrees, reading from left to right. The Fahrenheit thermometers read from about 94°F to about 107°F; Centigrade from about 34°C to about 42°C. In between the degree marks, there are smaller lines which represent either fifths (0.2) or tenths (0.1) of a degree.

You'll see that at the normal mark there's an arrow, or the letter 'N' or both. On Fahrenheit thermometers, this is at either 98.4 or 98.6. On Centigrade instruments, it's at either 36.9 or 37.

Before using the thermometer, make sure that the mercury column is down below the lower end of the scale. If it isn't, then shake it down. You do this by taking hold of the upper end of the thermometer (the one at the other end from the bulb) and snapping the instrument down sharply four or five times with a firm, wristy action.

Having shaken the thermometer down, put it in the child's mouth, with the bulb under his tongue.

In the case of younger children you'll have to use the armpit – just hold the child's arm gently but firmly across his chest or tummy so that the bulb is kept warm under his arm.

Although the instructions for many thermometers still say 'half minute', make sure the child always keeps the thermometer in the mouth or under the arm for at least two minutes. At the end of that time, withdraw it and read it. After reading it, shake it down, as before. Wash it in soap and cold water, and return it to its case.

A guide to what thermometer readings indicate is given on the opposite page.

TEMPER TANTRUMS

Unfortunately, many young children (especially in the age group one to three) are liable to throw tantrums. This is because the average toddler has very little control over his emotions.

So an occasional tantrum shouldn't be regarded as an ailment or disease. Just remember to keep calm yourself, so that the child does not let his rage feed on yours.

There is absolutely no point in slapping him, but neither should you give in to irrational demands. One of the world's top paediatricians advises that you should walk out of the room and leave him to work himself out of the temper, rather than stay and shout at him.

Obviously, there are some circumstances when you cannot walk away, and so you must just remain firm, quiet and as calm as possible.

Severe and recurrent problems with temper tantrums indicate that there are problems within the child and (most probably) the home situation, which could be helped by professional advice.

Begin by talking to your family doctor; who may well recommend that you have an initial chat with a psychologist. *(See also **Breath-holding Attacks**)*

TETANUS *(see Lockjaw)*

THRUSH

Thrush is an infection which affects both young babies and adult women (in the vagina).

It's caused by a fungus, and you may also hear it referred to as 'candida' or 'monilia'.

Thrush attacks the baby in the mouth, and gives her little sore patches inside her cheeks and on her tongue, which may make her cry a lot.

Characteristically, there are quite large white blobs of fungus material on the tongue and inside the cheeks. The doctor will prescribe anti-fungus medication to clear the condition up.

TICS

Tics are habitual sudden jerky movements. They often develop because a child is worried or is disturbed about something, for example a home or school problem. Tics may also be associated with cerebral palsy *(see **Cerebral Palsy**)*.

TONSILLITIS

Tonsillitis is inflammation of the tonsils, and it's caused by infection. The tonsils are small pieces of tissue situated at the back of the throat, one on either side. If you look in a child's mouth, you'll see them hanging down like a pair of rather baggy pink curtains.

The tonsils are there to trap many of the germs which children breathe in. The cells inside the tonsils attack the majority of these germs and soon render them completely harmless.

But trouble comes when, as so very often occurs, the tonsils are overwhelmed. When that happens, they usually become enlarged, red, inflamed and sometimes covered in pus.

The term tonsillitis covers anything from a very mild inflammation to a really roaring one.

Mild tonsillitis   Happily, most of the time this inflammation is mild.

All you may notice is that your child is a little off colour, and a bit grumpy. He may be off his food too, and have a very slight cough. You may decide to keep him away from school for a day or give him a little paracetamol. By the morning, he may be well on the road to recovery.

Severe tonsillitis   If you've got a child who has a severe bout of tonsillitis, he will feel absolutely rotten. He will be completely off his food, and if anybody tries to give him any he will vomit.

This is in fact a rather little-known hallmark of severe tonsillitis. He may also have a bit of a cough, swollen glands at the side of the neck, and a temperature.

This kind of tonsillitis needs medical advice. Treatment is obviously up to the individual doctor but she will probably prescribe antibiotics.

Otherwise the mainstays of treatment of severe tonsillitis are: to give plenty of fluids (preferably iced) but not food; and a little paracetamol in accordance with the doctor's instructions.

Try to keep the child's termperature down and don't over-heat her (see **Feverish Convulsions**).

Even children with the severest bout of tonsillitis will usually be better in a few days or so. Some may never have another really bad bout, while others will have an occasional one – or perhaps even two or three a year.

Tonsillectomy   This means removing the tonsils. Even today, many children have this done, but the operation is less common than it was.

Admittedly, some children do benefit from it but many others don't, and have gone through a very trying and traumatic procedure for nothing. Also, the operation does carry a very small, although a measurable, risk of death.

So, don't pressurise your doctor into arranging the operation. It may not be necessary.

TOOTHACHE
If you insist that your children clean their teeth thoroughly, two or three times a day, if you take them to the dentist twice a year, and if you reach a joint decision with your dentist about whether you want them to have fluoride painting or use fluoride tablets – then the risk of toothache occurring becomes very small indeed.

But if it happens, soak a bit of cotton wool in oil of cloves, and place it on the affected tooth. Give the child paracetamol and immediately seek the advice of a dentist.

TUBERCULOSIS (TB)

Tuberculosis is at present rare in most Western countries. However, occasional outbreaks do occur when youngsters are in contact with an adult who is coughing up TB germs.
The majority of cases of tuberculosis affect the lungs (pulmonary TB), but sometimes the bones and other organs are affected. A tuberculosis meningitis *(see **Meningitis**)* may also occur in some children.

Fortunately, early treatment of most types of TB is successful in nearly all cases.

TUMMY ACHE

Tummy ache in children is extremely common, and the first thing for any parent to understand is that in 99 cases out of 100 the tummy ache will go away by itself and cause no major problems.

However, every now and again a child develops abdominal pain because of some serious cause, such as appendicitis.

It is therefore important to have some rough idea of when a tummy ache is sufficiently bad to make it necessary to inform the doctor. In general, if a pain isn't distressing and has been going on for less than two hours, it's unlikely to be serious.

You should, however, be very suspicious of any abdominal pain associated with a temperature over 37.8°C (100°F).

Also, in a baby or young toddler you should be wary of severe pain which is accompanied by vomiting. This can be due to a serious condition in which the bowel telescopes up on itself (*see* **Intussusception**). In some cases, the baby passes blood-stained motions which rather resemble redcurrant jelly.

A pain in the abdomenal area may also be caused by an infection of the urinary tract *(see also **Urinary Problems**, **Colic in babies** and **Appendicitis**).*

Beware of pain which appears to be in a little boy's tummy, but which may be caused by a torsion (twisted testicle); this always needs an urgent operation.

Common Causes Most cases of tummy ache in childhood are just the result of indigestion or 'wind'. Also remarkably common are incidents of nervous tummy, in which the child responds to stress by producing a tummy ache. He is not making this up; he does feel discomfort in his tummy when he's frightened or worried

Tummy ache is very commonly associated with stomach germs which affect so many children and may cause diarrhoea *(see **Bowel Problems**).*

Another cause of tummy ache – but one which very few parents know about – is an infection in some part of the body, particularly in the throat.

Small glands inside the stomach swell up, as if in sympathy. This immediately produces abdominal discomfort and pain. The condition is called *Mesenteric adenitis*, which is not particularly serious; the discomfort will soon disappear as the infection clears.

Management   First, do not give your child a laxative – which is what many people think you should do. Take his temperature *(see **Taking Your Child's Temperature**)* and put him to bed.

If his temperature isn't raised, give him a nice, soothing hot water bottle on his tummy. (Not, of course, in the case of a baby – since babies can be burned by hot water bottles.)

Keep him on fluids only – and if the pain goes on for more than two or three hours, ask the doctor if the symptoms justify any further action.

Finally, don't make a big fuss about any tummy ache. There is an unfortunate, although an understandable, tendency for some children to notice the fact that abdominal pain can create anxiety in adults. They are then liable to make a fuss of the occasional bouts of discomfort in the abdomin which (after all) everybody gets from time to time.

URINARY INFECTIONS

Urinary infections are moderately common in young girls, but rare in young boys. This is mainly because males have a much longer urinary pipe (urethra), with its opening much further away from that rich source of germs, the anus.

The main symptoms of urinary infection are as follows: frequent urination; pain on passing water; fever; and possibly blood in the urine.

Always take your child to the doctor if she has symptoms suggesting urinary infection. The usual treatment is a course of antibiotics. Further investigations may be necessary, especially if the infection recurs.

URTICARIA

Often known as 'hives' or 'nettle rash', this is a common skin reaction which does actually look like the white lumpy appearance which people get when they're stung by nettles. But in urticaria, there are usually quite large raised, red or white, puffy areas of skin. A nettle sting produces fairly small spots.

Urticaria is a reaction to foreign agents such as foods, medicines, venom from insect bites, and inhaled matter. Often no cause can be identified.

Treatment is to remove the offending agent if possible and to give anti-histamine drugs.

VERRUCA

A verruca is a wart on the sole of the foot, caused by a virus. Vast numbers of children develop verrucas each year.

They are mildly infectious, so your child should not go around barefoot in changing rooms and swimming baths untill she is cured. If you buy one of those little verruca socks (from a sports shop), she'll be able to wear it at the pool and so not miss swimming.

There are special anti-verruca skin applications, but often they don't work very well. Sometimes it's better to have the wart burned away with cryotherapy (a very cold probe) or with a special acid, or removed by minor surgery.

VOMITING

The most valuable tip about vomiting for a parent to be aware of is this. If a child says she may vomit, believe her. Grab a large bowl or a stout plastic bag and (if possible) find the nearest lavatory. (Note: never allow your child to use a plastic bag without supervision.)

Here are some common causes of vomiting:

* Tummy infections caused by germs. These frequently cause diarrhoea as well *(see **Bowel Problems**)*

* Tonsillitis *(see **Tonsillitis**)*. When a child feels off-colour and vomits, the reason is often an infection of the tonsils

* Catarrh dripping down the throat

Some less common causes of vomiting include the following:

* Scarlet fever *(see **Scarlet Fever**)*

* Pneumonia *(see **Pneumonia**)*

* Whooping cough *(see **Whooping cough)***

* Psychological or hysterical vomiting

* Deliberate (i.e. self-induced) vomiting, for example to avoid school;

* Appendicitis, although the child with an acute appendix rarely vomits more than once or twice *(see **Appendicitis**)*

* Migraine *(see **Migraine**)*

WARTS
Warts are small benign growths on a child's skin, caused by a virus. They're mildly infectious and

children seem to be most vulnerable to them at play school and in their early school years. After that, they mainly seem to develop a resistance, although even elderly people get warts.

Medical treatment – which is not always very satisfactory – includes applying an anti-wart preparation on the skin, and wart removal with liquid nitrogen *(see also* **Verruca***)*

WASP STINGS *(see Stings)*

WAX (EAR)
Some children get a lot of wax in their ears, and others don't. This appears to be an inherited disorder. If your child's ear glands make a lot of wax all you must do is keep a watch for the symptom that suggest that wax is building up again, namely deafness (particularly after the child has been swimming). When this happens, take your child to the doctor, who will tell you if syringing is necessary. This takes about five min-utes, and shouldn't be painful, but the child may find this a bit alarming, especially if no
one has explained to her what the doctor or nurse is going to do.

The doctor can also tell you whether in the future it might be advisable to use a wax-dissolving preparation to prevent build-up of wax.

WHEEZING
This symptom suggests the possible presence of asthma *(see* **Asthma***)* or asthmatic bronchitis (see **Bronchitis**). So if your child wheezes, you should definaitely have his chest examined by your family doctor.

WHOOPING COUGH (Pertussis)
This used to be a very common (and often very serious) childhood illness. Happily, it has become rare in countries where the majority of infants are immunized against it.

The incubation period is about 12 days. The symptoms start with snuffling and a cough, and seem mild at first. But a week later, the poor child develops very violent bouts of coughing which half-choke him and often make him sick. Frequently, each bout finishes with an alarming crowing sound (the 'whoop').

Possible complications of whooping cough include lung, ear and brain problems. The infection can be difficult to treat, and may drag on for weeks. The advantages of immunization against it are obvious, despite the small risk of side-effects.

WORMS
Even in the most developed countries, children do get worms. If it happens, it's nothing to be ashamed of. There are various types of worms, including the following:

Threadworms These are common, giving rise to symptoms such as night-time itching round the child's anus, which is caused by the female threadworm emerging from his bottom to lay her eggs. This makes the child scratch his bottom, so the eggs get under his fingernails. From there, the eggs are easily transferred to his mouth, or to the mouths of other members of the family, or indeed friends.

You may be able to see the worms, looking like little white threads. Your doctor will probably want to treat the whole family with a drug which is called piperazine. In addition, cut the yougster's finernails short and make sure he always washes his hands before meals.

Roundworms These look like white earthworms. Understandably, children are very alarmed when they find they've passed one of these with a bowel motion. Take the child (and the worm, for identification) to the doctor; she will prescribe medication, and give advice about toilet hygiene. This is important, because roundworm eggs are spread when faecal material contaminates food, or when children play on contaminated soil.

A different type of roundworm *(Toxocara canis)* is caught from puppies and may cause childhood blindness. In fact, blindness from this cause is rare, but if you buy a puppy you should have it de-wormed regularly . Also, every parent should take care that their children do not come into contact with pet droppings.

Hookworms These are common in more tropical climates, including the southern United States. The infection is caught by walking in bare feet on ground which has been contaminated with human bowel motions containing hookworm larvae. The worm may cause anaemia, a cough, and other symptoms. Fortunately, drugs are very effective.

Tapeworms These are ribbon-shaped worms which your child could acquire through eating raw or badly-undercooked beef or pork. Symptoms: tummy ache, diarrhoea, weight loss. Effective drugs are available.